Table of Contents

INTRODUCTION

Healthy eating can be a fraught endeavor in this age of social media and click bait headlines. There is no lack of advice on what and how we should be eating from clean to paleo to keto and each enticement is often accompanied by a blockbuster health claim that a diet can cut your cancer risk in half or cure diabetes. Based on the idea that cancers grow in an acidic environment, the claim goes that eating a diet that is high in alkaline-based foods will create an internal environment that discourages the development of cancer. The alkaline diet is one in a string of evidence-based and non-evidence-based diet fads. The idea is to replace acid-forming foods with alkaline foods in order to balance your body's pH levels. Certain food components that can cause acidity in the body include protein, phosphate and sulfur. Acid and alkaline-based foods have a great impact on our bodies, our lungs and kidneys are largely responsible for controlling the pH of our blood, and it is imperative that it remain between 7.3 and 7.4 for survival. The pH of our urine can vary, with the kidney orchestrating what is eliminated to help maintain the balance. The actual pH in food doesn't determine a net effect on the body. Rather, the effect food has on the kidney, called the "potential renal acid load" or PRAL determines where they fit in the context of the acid-alkaline diet. For example, citrus fruits are acidic but are considered high alkaline foods because they have a low renal acid load. This may help clear up some confusion when looking at food lists for this diet. Looking at a list of foods along the acid/alkaline continuum, it is possible to consider that, over the long term, nutritional deficiencies may show up with those strictly adhering to an alkaline diet.

Likewise, it is conceivable that an eating pattern of high-PRAL (acidic) foods may lead to a depletion of alkaline buffers in our bodies with the largest reserve of these chemicals coming from our bones. Foods at the alkaline end of the spectrum are largely fruits and vegetables, and time-honored nutrition advice tells us that a plant-based diet is best for our health. However, a healthy eating pattern also includes lean meats and whole grains, which fall on the acidic end of the spectrum. Recommendations aren't based on the acidity or alkalinity of the foods but rather the fact that these foods are rich in vitamins, minerals, phyto nutrients and fiber. Patients with cancer, especially those undergoing treatment, are advised to maintain their current body weight with adequate calories and protein. While it wouldn't necessarily be unsafe for cancer patients to follow the alkaline diet, they would need to ensure that their protein and calorie needs are being met and should consult with a dietitian for nutrition optimization. Optimal health includes maintaining a healthy body weight, regular physical activity, quality sleep, stress reduction and social connections.

ALKALINE DIET

The alkaline diet is also known as the acid-alkaline diet or alkaline ash diet. The alkaline diet is said to improve health and fight serious diseases like cancer. Although the diet is actually quite healthy in essence, there is no evolutionary evidence or human physiological evidence to support some of the many health claims. The reason the diet is a healthy one is because it encourages the consumption of natural unprocessed plant-based foods and lots of fruits and vegetables. But acids, such as amino acids and fatty acids, are actually an extremely important part of any diet in people who don't have tolerance to them, and should not be cut out. Food components that leave an acidic ash include protein, phosphate, and sulfur, while alkaline components include calcium, magnesium, and Acidic: meat, poultry, fish, dairy, eggs, grains, alcohol. The alkaline diet and its possible connections with cancer is a controversial subject. However, researchers do agree that what you eat can impact your cancer risk. The connection between pH changes and cancer lies in the amount of acid in the system. The body must remain at a pH level of around 7.35 to optimally transport oxygen. If something like an illness causes a pH imbalance, the body naturally corrects itself using substances that neutralize acids. Problems can happen when a person eats a high-acid diet – such as eating a lot of processed foods, junk foods, and sodas.

Consistently eating high-acid foods can force the body to work harder to maintain an optimal pH balance. This can eventually lead to a depletion in the body's natural alkaline reserves, and a more acidic overall pH level. If this happens, the body releases excess acids into the tissues, which can begin to deteriorate. Without reversing the process, the person could be at risk of cell death or abnormal cell growth. Abnormal cells are malignant and can grow indefinitely (cancer cells).

What you eat can have an effect on your cancer risk. Eating foods that naturally help your body maintain a healthy pH can balance out your system and help you reduce the odds of cancer cell development. Caring for your body properly with whole foods can boost your system's natural ability to heal itself. Rather than working hard to balance out the acidity of processed foods, your body can focus on other things.

Neutral: natural fats, starches, and sugars

Alkaline: fruits, nuts, legumes, and vegetables

The term P.H means a measurement of how acidic or alkaline something is. This is an important foundation of the alkaline diet, and the ideas behind it. PH is a measure of acidity/alkalinity on a scale of 0-14. Seven is neutral, with anything above that alkaline and anything below that acid

Alkaline-ash foods or Acid-ash foods: This is based on the ash that remains after the combustion of foods under laboratory conditions.

Regular pH levels in the body

The pH value ranges from 0–14:

Acidic: 0.0–6.9

Neutral: 7.0

Alkaline (or basic): 7.1–14.0

Many proponents of this diet suggest that people monitor the pH of their urine to ensure that it is alkaline (over 7) and not acidic (below 7). However, it's important to note that pH varies greatly within your body. While some parts are acidic, others are alkaline there is no set level.

The stomach is loaded with hydrochloric acid, giving it a pH of 2–3.5, which is highly acidic. This acidity is necessary to break down food. On the other hand, human blood is always slightly alkaline, with a pH of 7.36–7.44. When the blood pH falls out of the normal range, it can be fatal if left untreated. However, this only happens during certain disease states, such as ketoacidosis caused by diabetes, starvation, or alcohol intake.

Food that affects the pH of urine and not the blood

It's critical for the health that the pH of the blood remains constant. If it were to fall outside of the normal range, the cells would stop working and this can cause death very quickly if untreated. For this reason, the body has many effective ways to closely regulate its pH balance. This is known as acid-base homeostasis.

 It is nearly impossible for food to change the pH value of blood in healthy people, although tiny fluctuations can occur within the normal range. However, food can change the pH value of ones urine though the effect is somewhat variable.Excreting acids in the urine is one of the main ways the body regulates its blood PH.

If a large stake is consume, the urine will be more acidic several hours later as the body removes the metabolic waste from the system.Therefore, urine pH is a poor indicator of overall body pH and general health.It can also be influenced by factors other than ones diet.

Acid-forming foods and osteoporosis

Osteoporosis is a progressive bone disease characterized by a decrease in bone mineral content. It's particularly common among postmenopausal women and can drastically increase the risk of fractures.

Many alkaline-diet proponents believe that to maintain a constant blood pH, the body takes alkaline minerals, such as calcium from your bones, to buffer the acids from the acid-forming foods taken.

According to this theory, acid-forming diets, such as the standard Western diet, will cause a loss in bone mineral density. This theory is known as the "acid-ash hypothesis of osteoporosis." However, this theory ignores the function of the kidneys, which are fundamental to removing acids and regulating body pH. The kidneys produce bicarbonate ions that neutralize acids in the blood, enabling the body to closely manage blood PH. The respiratory system is also involved in controlling blood pH. When bicarbonate ions from the kidneys bind to acids in the blood, they form carbon dioxide, which we breathe out, and water, which we pee out.

The acid-ash hypothesis also ignores one of the main drivers of osteoporosis loss in the protein collagen from bone. Ironically, this loss of collagen is strongly linked to low levels of two acids orthosilicic acid and ascorbic acid, or vitamin C in our diet.

We should keep in mind that scientific evidence linking dietary acid to bone density or fracture risk is mixed. While many observational studies have found no association, others have detected a significant link. Clinical trials, which tend to be more accurate, have concluded that acid-forming diets have no impact on calcium levels in the body. These diets improve bone health by increasing calcium retention and activating the IGF-1 hormone, which stimulates the repair of muscle and bone As such, a high-protein, acid-forming diet is likely linked to better bone health not worse.

Acidity and cancer

Many people argue that cancer only grows in an acidic environment and can be treated or even cured with an alkaline diet. However, comprehensive reviews on the relationship between diet-induced acidosis or increased blood acidity caused by diet and cancer concluded that there is no direct ;

First, food doesn't significantly influence blood Ph. Second, even if you assume that food could dramatically alter the pH value of blood or other tissues, cancer cells are not restricted to acidic environments.

In fact, cancer grows in normal body tissue, which has a slightly alkaline pH of 7.4. Many experiments have successfully grown cancer cells in an alkaline environment. And while tumors grow faster in acidic environments, tumors create this acidity themselves. It is not the acidic environment that creates cancer cells, but cancer cells that create the acidic environment.

That is, there is no link between an acid-forming diet and cancer. Cancer cells also grow in alkaline environments.

Acid and Alkaline Foods

When foods containing protein are metabolized, most proteins release acid (H+/hydrogen ions) because of the metabolism of amino acids. The amount of acid depends on which amino acids are present: some amino acids are neutral, some acidic, and some alkaline. Lysine, arginine, and histidine are acidic, and when metabolized in the liver generate hydrochloric acid (plus glucose and urea). The amino acids, cysteine and methionine, contain sulfur and are converted to sulfuric acid:

Arginine+$\rightarrow$H++Cl−+Glucose + Urea

Cysteine→2H++SO4−+Glucose + Urea

Most F&V when metabolized produce alkali which neutralizes the acid. F&V contain organic acids such as citric acid and organic salts, for example, potassium citrate. The organic acids, when metabolized, produce equal amounts of hydrogen and base ions, but the organic salts contain base ions but no hydrogen and, therefore, "mop up" hydrogen ions on their metabolism to carbon dioxide and water. This reduces the acid load:

Potassiumcitrate→Citrate3−+3K+

Citrate3−+3H++4.5O2→6CO2+4H2O

Foods which contain phosphate, whether naturally or from food additives, can add acid to the diet. The acidity depends not on the phosphate anion but on the cation to which it is attached and the pH of the food. For example, phosphoric acid (H3PO4) in cola drinks is acidic as H+ is released, whereas the food additive trisodium phosphate (Na3PO4) is alkaline and will remove H+.

H3PO4→H++H2PO41−(excretedasH2PO41−intheurine)

Na3PO4+2H+→NaH2PO4+2Na+→H2PO41−(inurine)

Fats and sugars, unless incompletely metabolized, have only a small effect on acid–base balance.

Ancestral diets and acidity

Examining the acid-alkaline theory from both an evolutionary and scientific perspective reveals discrepancies.

One study estimated that 87% of pre-agricultural humans ate alkaline diets and formed the central argument behind the modern alkaline diet. More recent research approximates that half of pre-agricultural humans ate net alkaline-forming diets, while the other half ate net acid-forming diets.

Know well that our remote ancestors lived in vastly different climates with access to diverse foods. In fact, acid-forming diets were more common as people moved further north of the equator, away from the tropics.

Although around half of hunter-gatherers were eating a net acid-forming diet, modern diseases are believed to have been much less common.

Current studies suggest that about half of ancestral diets were acid-forming, especially among people who lived far from the equator.

SUMMARY

The alkaline diet is quite healthy, encouraging a high intake of fruits, vegetables, and healthy plant foods while restricting processed junk foods.

However, the notion that the diet boosts health because of its alkalizing effects is suspect. These claims haven't been proven by any reliable human studies. Some studies suggest positive effects in a very small subset of the population. Specifically, a low-protein alkalizing diet may benefit people with chronic kidney disease.

In general, the alkaline diet is healthy because it's based on whole and unprocessed foods. No reliable evidence suggests it has anything to do with pH levels.

There is general agreement amongst natural healers and medical professionals alike, that changing a cancer patient's diet is extremely helpful when someone is confronted with a cancer diagnosis. The goal of an alkaline diet for cancer is to achieve an optimal balance between acid-forming and alkaline-forming foods. The alkaline diet for cancer greatly reduces the strain on the bodys acid-detoxification systems. The alkaline diet, which is primarily plant-based and avoids sugar, dairy, wheat and other high-gluten grains as well as an excess consumption of fruits, while emphasizing fresh vegetables and vegetable juices along with cruciferous vegetables and greens, changes the body's intracellular pH to come close to the ideal blood pH of 7.3/7.41 — a key metabolic accomplishment on the path to longevity whether you have cancer or not! An alkaline diet based on vegetables and fruits, creates a less-than-optimal environment for cancer proliferation, while at the same time strengthens the immune function and supports healthy cells in the body through improved nutrition.

ALKALINE WATER

Alkaline water is bottled water with a higher pH level than typical drinking water. Alkaline water is the opposite of acidic water. It has a higher pH level than plain water. The pH of water is neutral, around pH 7. Chemicals and gases can change this to make it more acidic or more alkaline.

The pH of water is around 7, but some people say it may be more healthful to drink water that is alkaline. Rainwater's pH is slightly below neutral, because there is carbon dioxide from the air, and this increases acidity. Acidic substances have a pH of below 7.0, down to zero. The pH of vinegar is around pH 3, lemon juice around pH 2, and battery acid around pH 1. Alkaline substances have a pH up to 14. Baking soda's pH is between pH 8 and 9 and milk of magnesia is between pH 10 and 11. Water can be high or low in pH, but if it is too high or too low, it can have adverse effects. Water that is too alkaline has a bitter taste. It can cause deposits that encrust pipes and appliances. Highly acidic water may corrode metals or even dissolve them.

Alkaline water has become popular in recent years due to a belief that it may benefit health. Some research has been done on the effects of alkaline intake on bones. A study published in Bone found an effect on bone resorption. Bone resorption is the process where old bone cells are broken down and replaced by new ones, Less bone resorption and more mineral density result in better bone strength.

Acid Reflux

Reflux disease is when the contents of the stomach, which are acidic, splash back up the food pipe. Acid reflux that keeps happening for a long time can cause damage and a disease known as gastroesophageal reflux disease, or GERD.

A study published in Annals of Otology, Rhinology & Laryngology found that drinking alkaline water might be worth further study as a supplement to other treatments for reflux disease. It found that alkaline water at pH 8.8 stops an enzyme that is connected to reflux disease. It also appeared to reduce the acidity of the stomach contents.

Moreover, stomach acid exists for a purpose. It kills bacteria and other pathogens, and it helps our bodies to digest food and absorb nutrients.

The Role of the Kidney in Maintaining Acid–Base Balance

The kidney helps maintain acid-base balance by 3 main mechanisms: (1) excretion of acid, (2) neutralization of acid and (3) excretion of anions.

Excretion of Acid

Dietary acid has to be excreted by the kidney. Phosphate is the primary buffer in the urine and accepts $H+$ ions ($HPO42- + H+ \rightarrow H2PO41-$). The quantity of phosphate excreted is mainly dependent on dietary phosphate and usually varies between 10 and 45 mmol/day.

 About 80% of the phosphate filtered at the glomerulus is in the monohydrate form ($HPO42-$) and will remove $H+$ ions. The remaining phosphate is already present in the diprotic form ($H2PO41-$) and therefore unable to remove additional hydrogen. When the pH of the urine falls, creatinine, urate, and other anions filtered at the glomerulus act as urinary buffers, removing additional hydrogen ions. Acid excreted with phosphate and other urinary buffers is known as titratable acid (TA).

Neutralization of Acid

Historically, it was believed that ammonia was also a urinary buffer accepting $H+$ ($NH3 + H+ \rightarrow NH4+$) and thus increasing acid excretion. However, it is now recognized that the remaining acid is not excreted but only neutralized within the kidney and ammonium is a by-product of this.

Neutralization of acid occurs through the metabolism of glutamine. In the proximal tubule of the kidney, glutamine is taken from the blood stream and broken down to alpha-ketoglutarate (AKG2−) and ammonium. AKG2− consumes 2 H+ on its metabolism to glucose, thus reducing the acid load and the ammonium is excreted into the lumen of the nephron:

Glutamine→Glutamate→AKG2−+2NH4+

AKG2−+2H+→Glucose(orCO2+H2O)

This ammonium is recycled in the loop of Henle via a medullary shunt, a mechanism that allows fine tuning of acid excretion and may allow additional distal [H+] to be excreted without lowering the pH of the urine. When the diet is very acidic, there are small increases in TA, limited by the amount of phosphate in the diet, but significant increases in ammonium excretion which can increase 10-fold.

This gives flexibility to the body allowing it to neutralize large acid loads. However, ammonium excretion takes several days to maximize as glutamine uptake is stimulated in the proximal tubule together with increased production of the enzymes converting glutamine to AKG.

Excretion of Anions

Some organic anions like citrate, oxalate, and urate are excreted in the urine, and this is a loss of alkali to the body as some of these anions, for example, citrate could have been metabolized to alkaline end products. Others, like urate and oxalate, are end products of metabolism. The amount of organic anion excreted is estimated for body surface area and is part of NEAP calculations. Organic anion excretion is considered to be fairly constant, although recent studies suggest significant increases of organic anions occur with increased intakes of protein and certain F&V. When the urine is very acidic, some of these anions will be excreted in the urine with H+as organic acids and will be measured as part of TA excretion. The total amount of acid excreted and neutralized by the kidney can be measured directly from 24-hour urine samples and is known as net acid excretion (NAE).

$NAE(mEq/d)=NH4++TA-HCO3-$ When eating an acidic diet, the amount of bicarbonate excreted is negligible to conserve alkali.

Alkaline Diet Food List

The diet is organized around the pH of individual foods. Some versions are less strict, meaning they may allow grains for their health benefits despite their slightly acidic pH. But generally, if you're following the alkaline diet, you'll want to follow the food list below, steering clear of the acidic foods, limiting or avoiding the neutral foods, and focusing on the alkaline foods.

Acidic Foods to Avoid

Meat (especially corned beef, canned lunch meat, turkey, veal, and lean beef)

Poultry

Fish

Cottage cheese

Milk

Cheese (especially Parmesan cheese, reduced-fat cheddar, and hard cheeses)

Yogurt

Ice cream

Eggs (the egg yolk in particular)

Grains (brown rice, rolled oats, spaghetti, cornflakes, white rice, rye bread, whole-wheat bread)

Alcohol

Soda

Lentils

Peanuts and walnuts

Other packaged, processed food

Neutral Foods to Limit

Natural fats such as olive oil, cream, butter, and milk

Starches

Sugars

Alkaline Foods to Eat

Fruit

Unsweetened fruit juices

Raisins

Black currants

Vegetables (especially spinach)

Potatoes

Wine

Mineral soda water

Soy food

Legumes

Seeds

Nuts

Some foods are more alkaline than others based on their acid content. People who follow an alkaline diet try to consume foods that are higher in pH levels, with the goal of increasing their bodies' alkalinity to ward off cancer cells. The following foods make up most of what someone practicing an alkaline diet would eat, organized by pH level.

High alkaline content:

• Mineral water

• Ginger tea

• Blackberries

• Raspberries

• Strawberries

• Tangerines

• Limes

• Papaya

• Pineapple

• Melons

• Kale

• Mustard greens

• Sweet potatoes

• Asparagus

• Onions

• Sea salt

• Ginger roots

• Chestnuts

• Parsley

• Pumpkin seeds

Medium alkaline content:

• Grapefruit juice

- Pineapple juice

- Apple cider vinegar

- Apples

- Grapes

- Raisins

- Blueberries

- Oranges

- Apricots

- Grapefruit

- Avocados

- Green olives

- Bananas

- Lemons

- Artichokes

- Eggplants

- Squash

- Zucchinis

- Bell peppers

- Broccoli

- Cabbage

- Garlic

- Basil

- Cashews

- Cilantro

- Cinnamon

Low alkaline content:

- Apple juice

- Grape juice

- Orange juice

- Herbal teas

- Coconuts

- Carrots

- Cucumbers

- Snow peas

- Cauliflower

- Brussels sprouts

- Mushrooms

- Ghee

• Oils (olive, flax, coconut, avocado, cod liver)

• Almonds

• Oatmeal

• Quinoa

• Wild rice

• Unsweetened granola

• Sesame/sunflower seeds

• Bay leaves

• Almonds

• Cayenne pepper

• Rice syrup

ALKALINE DIET MEAL PLAN

1. Green Pea and Avocado SpreadGreen Pea and Avocado Spread

Source: Green Pea and Avocado Spread

Green Pea and Avocado Spread has the sweet, refreshing taste of green peas combined with creamy avocado. Not only is it super healthy, it's also alkaline and super-versatile.

2. Onion and Bell Pepper Masala Onion and Bell Pepper Masala

Source: Onion and Bell Pepper Masala

Onion and Bell Pepper Masala recipe is a deliciously spicy and complex-tasting addition to any alkaline-friendly dinner table.

3. Raw Vegan Melt away Balls Raw Vegan Melt away Balls

Source: Raw Vegan Melt away Balls

Raw Vegan Melt away Balls can be eaten for breakfast or as a snack throughout the day.

4. Broccoli Mushroom Rotini Casserole

Source: Broccoli Mushroom Rotini Casserole

Vegetables like broccoli, Brussels sprouts, cabbage, and cauliflower are alkaline-promoting foods. So try this delicious Broccoli Mushroom Rotini Casserole for the perfect dinner.

5. Kale and Golden Beet SaladKale and Golden Beet Salad

Source: Kale and Golden Beet Salad

Greens like kale, spinach, lettuce, and collard greens are great alkaline foods to incorporate with Salad will make the perfect light lunch or side dish.

6. Spanakopita: Greek Spinach PieSpanakopita: Greek Spinach Pie

Source: Spanakopita: Greek Spinach Pi

Greek Spinach Pie has the feta from the traditional recipe removed, in favor of healthier ingredients.

7. High Protein Spinach and Rice Balls

Source: High Protein Spinach and Rice Balls

For another dish packed with spinach, try this High Protein Spinach and Rice Balls recipe. They're easy and fun to make and also great way to get your greens in, kids will love them.

8. Lime and Coconut Panna CottaLime and Coconut Panna Cotta

Source: Lime and Coconut Panna Cotta

Lemon and limes are acidic but they become alkaline within the body. This Lime and Coconut Panna Cotta has a light, mild lime flavor which still manages to overpower the coconut.

9. Creamy Lemon Herb Dressing

Source: Creamy Lemon Herb Dressing

You can also use this Creamy Lemon Herb on your spinach salad, for the ultimate alkalized dish.

10. Minced Tempeh Salad With Lemongrass, Sesame, and Cashews

Source: Minced Tempeh Salad with Lemongrass, Sesame, and Cashews

Nuts, such as almonds, cashews, macadamia, and chestnuts are another great alkalizing food group. Minced Tempeh Salad With Lemongrass, Sesame, and Cashews is easy to add into your diet.

11. Energency Protein Bars

Source: Energency Protein Bars

These Energency Protein Bars are a perfect way to get some nuts into your diet, and are easy to take with you on the go or to eat on your ride home.

12. Traditional 'Beef' Stew Recipe

Source: Traditional 'Beef' Stew Recipe

Root vegetables include sweet potatoes, potatoes, yams, and carrots. These alkaline vegetables are easy to incorporate. This Traditional 'Beef' Stew Recipe will warm your entire soul.

13. Lentil-Stuffed Potato CakesLentil-Stuffed Potato Cakes

Source: Lentil-Stuffed Potato Cakes

 Lentil-Stuffed Potato Cakes include 2 alkaline foods; lentils and potatoes. Beside being really, really good for you, they taste really, really delicious too.

14. Savory Sweet Potato Breakfast BowlSavory Sweet Potato Breakfast Bowl

Source: Savory Sweet Potato Breakfast Bowl

 Savory Sweet Potato Breakfast Bowl recipe is a great way to add sweet potatoes in for breakfast. It's also very, very easy to make.

15. Thai Green Vegetable CurryThai Green Vegetable Curry

Source: Thai Green Vegetable Curry

For the perfect lunch, Green Vegetable Curry bowl is good. For extra protein, you can add tofu or a variety of different beans.

BENEFIT OF ALKALINE DIET

Alkaline diets reduce a person's consumption of fatty and processed meats, and they encourage people to eat more fruits and vegetables. This offers several health benefits.

Here are some of the benefits that alkaline has;

Promoting weight loss

Many strategies can help people lose weight. Ultimately, weight loss depends on consuming fewer calories than one burn. Diets lower in fat and calories may promote weight loss, but only when a person remains physically active and eats a healthful diet with variety. An alkaline diet tends to be low in calories, so it may help people lose weight.

Improving kidney health

Raising urine pH may improve health for some people. According to a 2017 study, the typical diet of people in the United States is very acidic. This can challenge the kidneys. For people with kidney disease, a lower-acid diet may improve symptoms or even slow the course of the disease. For most people with chronic kidney disease, there is no need to follow a specific alkaline diet. Instead, simply reducing protein, such as milk, meat, and cheese, may help.

Preventing cancer

Some proponents of this diet claim that it can reverse cancer or support chemotherapy. There is no scientific evidence supporting these claims, and no studies have performed direct tests on this claim.

However, significant evidence from a 2010 study suggests that reducing meat consumption and eating more fruits, vegetables, and whole grains might prevent cancer. The study looked at data from the 2010 European Prospective Investigation into Cancer and Nutrition. It found that consuming vitamin C, vitamin A, fiber, and a Mediterranean-style diet might reduce cancer risk.

The American Cancer Society (ACS) recommend a diet similar, but not identical, to an alkaline diet. The ACS advise avoiding processed foods, soft drinks, and many high-fat foods. Instead, it is more beneficial to eat a diet rich in fruit, vegetables, and whole grains.

Treating or preventing heart disease

In the U.S., heart disease is the leading cause of death. Lifestyle factors including poor nutrition and low activity levels are major contributors.

An alkaline diet may naturally raise levels of growth hormone, but the research is preliminary and inconclusive. Research finds that growth hormone supports body composition and lowers heart disease risk factors. Alkaline diets also tend to be low in fat and calories, naturally promoting a healthy body weight and lowering heart disease risk factors. They also reduce or eliminate red and processed meats, removing a major contributor to heart disease from the diet.

Improving growth hormone levels

Better heart health is just one potential benefit of having higher growth hormone levels. Improving growth hormone levels may also promote better brain functioning, particularly memory and cognition.

Some evidence suggests that growth hormone improves overall quality of life. However, the evidence linking an alkaline diet to increases in growth hormone levels is weak. Some studies have shown that correcting a highly acidic environment with specific supplements such as bicarbonate can promote alkalinity, but this does not necessarily mean that an alkaline diet has similar benefits.

Cure back pain

A small amount of research suggests that supplementing the diet with alkaline minerals might help with symptoms of back pain. This research does not directly test the benefits of an alkaline diet, so it is uncertain whether alkaline foods might help with chronic pain.

Preventing osteoporosis

Osteoporosis is a major risk factor for bone fractures, especially in older people and females. Some proponents of this diet say that it reduces the amount of calcium lost in urine, and that this lowers osteoporosis risk. However, no scientific evidence supports this claim.

That said, eating more fruits and vegetables may improve bone health. Alkaline diets are rich in these foods. They also tend to be low in protein, which supports bone and muscle health. It is unlikely, therefore, that an alkaline diet can prevent osteoporosis. Extremely low-protein alkaline diets may also be an osteoporosis risk factor. A better strategy is to eat more lean proteins, fruits, and vegetables.

Promoting healthy muscles

People tend to lose muscle mass as they age. This increases a person's risk of falls and fractures, and it may also contribute to weakness and chronic pain. A 2013 study offers preliminary evidence that an alkaline diet may improve muscle health.

Researchers examined 2,689 females in a long-term twin study. They found a small but significant increase in muscle mass among females following a more alkaline diet.

A diet rich in variety is the most healthful option. People should aim for a diet that includes a range of different proteins, grains, fruits, vegetables, vitamins, and minerals.

Removing any single food group or type of food from a diet can make it more difficult for a person to be healthy. Very low-protein alkaline diets may help people lose weight, but they may also increase the risk of other issues, such as weak bones and muscles.

People who wish to try an alkaline diet should ensure that they eat enough protein. Those who are able to eat enough protein on an alkaline diet can safely try it.

While the alkaline diet does not actually change blood pH, it can help people eat a wide range of healthful foods, improving overall health. People with serious medical conditions or a history of nutritional problems should consult a doctor before trying this diet.

Principle Ways of Taking Alkaline Diet

1) Eat a Wide Variety of Fresh, Quality Whole Foods

First consideration for eating the Alkaline Way is to eat predominantly whole foods (better even when grown organically or biodynamically). This is the basis of eating the Alkaline Way. Focus should be on eating plant-based, what we call "lively" foods including fresh vegetables and fruits, lightly toasted nuts and seeds, lightly steamed vegetables, sprouts of grains and beans, fermented foods, freshly squeezed fruit juices, and vegetable juices. These foods retain active enzymes that enhance digestion.

For maximum health benefit, eat a wide variety of whole foods. Eating the same foods repeatedly limits digestive and nutritional variety and also increases the likelihood of becoming reactive to those foods if digestion is weak, stressed, or compromised. Diversify your choices for those foods that are easy for you to digest, assimilate, and eliminate. Experiment with new flavors and often get a health bonus as well.

2) Eat 60-80% Alkaline-Forming Foods

Principle two is to select predominately alkaline foods. If you are already in good health, we recommend eating at least 60% alkaline-forming foods. If your immune system is compromised or reacting to something or your health needs to be restored in any way, we suggest an 80% alkalinizing diet, to help calm your immune system and support digestion.

Refer to the Food & Chemical Effects on Acid/Alkaline Body Chemical Balance chart to learn about acid-forming and alkaline-forming foods. Those foods that are alkalinizing and that you most enjoy will become the cornerstones of your shopping lists—the staples of your personal healthy eating plan.

You will refer to this chart frequently when creating shopping lists.

3) Eat Immune System Friendly Foods

The third Alkaline Way principle for healthy eating is to avoid any foods to which your immune system reacts.

Most overweight people lose weight effortlessly (even if they eat more calories) and enhance metabolism when they substitute nonreactive foods for those that cause them reactions and eat the Alkaline Way. Conversely, many underweight people gain healthy weight, because protein synthesis and repair are enhanced through a health-promoting diet.

4) Eat 60-70% Plant-Based, Complex Carbs; 15-20% Protein; 15-20% Healthy Fat

Our fourth Alkaline Way principle encourages a healthy ratio of complex carbohydrates to proteins to fats.

Recommended Ratios:

* 60–70% of calories from whole food (plant-based) complex carbohydrates

* 15–20% of calories from protein

* 15–20% of calories from healthy fats (including plenty of omega-3 fats)

Whole Food (Plant-based) Complex Carbohydrates:

Unless your health care practitioner instructs you differently, your Alkaline Way eating plan should be rich in complex carbohydrates from vegetables, whole grains, and legumes (beans, peas and lentils), as well as seasonings, spices, and herbs. These should comprise about 60-70% of your food intake.

Quality Protein:

Proteins should be approximately 15-20% of your total calorie intake. Approximately 50 to 60 grams of protein per day is a good amount for most people. Sources of protein may include organic eggs and dairy products, whey protein, as well as deep cold-water fish such as mackerel, sardines, tuna, herring, and salmon. Additional protein sources include nuts and seeds, sprouts, nutritional yeast, blue-green algae, miso, and mushrooms. You may also create "complimentary proteins" (by pairing grains with beans, and/or gains with dairy). Protein requirements may be higher if you are pregnant, recovering from chronic illness, exercise intensively, or have other specific needs. Be sure to work with your health care practitioner if you have special circumstances.

Healthy Fats:

Fat should be 15-20% of your daily calories. Be sure to focus on healthy omega-3 essential fats, which enhance your body's energy production, protein production, and tissue repair. Food-based sources of protective omega-3 essential fats are found in fresh nuts and seeds as well as cold-pressed organic oils such as avocados, olive oil, safflower, flaxseed, walnut, sesame, peanut, and pure deep-sea fish oils.

Other sources include borage, black currant, grape-seed and evening primrose oils, and Udo's oil™. Unless you eat line-caught, oily, deep-water fish more than three times per week, omega-3 supplements are recommended. When selecting omega 3 supplements ensure they are obtained from uncontaminated sources and are not contaminated or oxidized during processing. PERQUE EPA/DHA Guard is the recommended Alkaline Way omega-3 supplement.

Food Pairing to Create Complete Proteins:

Unlike animal proteins, plant proteins lack some essential amino acids. By pairing foods based on the amino acid supplied, you are able to obtain a complete protein. For example, brown rice and cooked beans each lack an important amino acid and are incomplete proteins when eaten alone; however, when eaten together, they complement each other and provide a source of complete protein.

Some food pairings that make a "complete protein":

* Beans and rice or corn

* Legumes with grains, nuts, seeds or dairy

* Grains with dairy

* Dairy with nuts, seeds and legumes

As described in Francis Moore Lappé's bestseller Diet for a Small Planet and updated more recently by Michael Polen, complementary proteins are as ancient as agriculture. These are reflected in many contemporary dishes, including:

* Corn, beans, and rice

* Rice and Indian dal

* Brown rice with chopped walnuts

* Bulgur wheat dishes with garbanzo beans

* Whole wheat bread with almond butter

Avoid Trans Fats and Hydrogenated Oils

"Trans" fatty acids are handled by the body as if they were natural saturated fats like butter or coconut oil, but these types of fat are more harmful. Trans fats cross the placenta, are stored in fetal tissue, and can cause long- term problems with cell membrane function. Unfortunately, "trans" fats are found everywhere—in fried foods such as French fries, in many processed foods, and in everything from conventional name-brand cooking oils to bakery goods and candy.

Use unsaturated, non-hydrogenated "expeller-pressed" and preferably organic or biodynamic oils such as olive, grapeseed, coconut, and peanut, along with exotic oils such as avocado, almond and mustard seed. Avoid solid cooking fats such as margarine, hydrogenated vegetable oils, lard and Crisco. You'll also want to pass up deep-fried fast food.

Hydrogenated oils can interfere with liver enzymes and are associated with higher cholesterol levels. These artificial oils can also have a negative effect on immune function and are known to promote certain types of tumors.

5) Include Probiotic and Fermented (Cultured) Foods and Drinks

The fifth principle of The Alkaline Way is to make a habit of consuming a wide range of probiotic (cultured or fermented) foods and drinks. The term probiotic means promoting life. A healthy gastrointestinal tract is home to a plentiful variety of beneficial (probiotic) bacteria responsible for keeping our bodies and immune systems in balance. Poor diet, stress, illness, and antibiotics can deplete these beneficial bacteria, giving pathogens free rein to proliferate. We consume probiotics to colonize the gut with beneficial bacteria.

Consuming probiotics in food or drink form is ideal, since this provides the highest levels and variety of probiotics. Additionally, probiotic supplements, such as PERQUE Digesta Guard, are highly beneficial. We recommend 2-4 capsules with each meal.

Some Probiotic-rich Foods and Drinks

* Kombucha (fermented tea)

* Kefir (fermented milk)

* Yogurt (dairy or nondairy, with live cultures)

* Sauerkraut (fermented cabbage)

* Kimchi (a spicy fermented cabbage common in the Korean diet)

* Tempeh (fermented soybeans)

* Microalgae (freeze dried)

* Hatcho Miso soup

* Pickles

* Olives

* Natto (a fermented soybean)

6) Eat Plenty of Fiber and Water

Plentiful water and fiber intake make up the sixth Alkaline Way principle. Americans, as a whole, consume far too little water and food fiber. Traditional cultures that remain free of Western degenerative diseases consume 40-100 grams of dietary fiber daily from whole, lively foods. By contrast, Americans typically consume 10 grams.

We recommend a daily fiber intake of at least 40 grams. The beneficial "roughage" from fiber makes the stool bulky and soft and helps to maintain a shorter transit time—the time from food consumption to waste elimination. Adequate fiber encourages wastes to be eliminated easily and comfortably on a regular basis. Keeping your body clean and clear means it is less likely that toxic waste matter will be reabsorbed back into circulation.

A healthy transit time ranges from 12–18 hours. This reduces the opportunity for unhealthy bacteria and yeast to dominate in the body.

The Importance of Water

Plentiful water intake is key to health—especially when consuming a high-fiber diet. Waterhelps fiber do its job of efficiently moving wastes through the body, and every system of the body depends on water to function. When following The Alkaline Way program, we recommend consuming at least one 8-ounce glass of purified water 8 times daily. For every 5-8 ounces of caffeinated beverages, add a glass of water. Take a rest from drinking water 20-30 minutes before and after meals to assist the body's digestive process. If you must drink at these times, make it small amounts of room temperature or hot water (or healthy tea)—cold water can really slow down digestion. Fresh lemon juice, lime juice, and/or ginger act as digestive aids and alkaline enhancers while enhancing the taste of water.

7) Eat Healthier Food Combinations

Smart food combining is an integral component of the Alkaline Way and is our final principle. The way we combine foods together during mealtime can have a tremendous impact on digestion, and therefore overall health. Just as the typical American diet is unhealthy, the American meal—usually represented as meat (protein) and potatoes (starch)—combines foods in the least effective manner.

The art of healthy food combining is an important aspect of balanced nutrition, and lessens wear and tear on the digestive system. Pay extra close attention to food combining if you are prone to any digestive discomforts (acid reflux, bloating, leaky gut, heartburn, irritable bowel, diverticulosis, or other digestive problems).

While this guide can't cover every facet of optimal food combining, we encourage you to read about and research healthy food combining. The main principles of healthy food combining are simplicity and compatibility. There are some diets out there that may be suitable to what you're wanting to do, such as the Shibboleth Diet and others.

However, not all diets are ideal. While other diets like the ABC Diet don't provide long-lasting, healthy impact, the Alkaline Way gives you what you need to live a healthy life.

PRINCIPLE ADVICE TO FOLLOW-UP BY A CANCER PATIENT

Before treatment one should start focusing on healthy food habits which may help to increase your energy. To prepare yourself and your home for your nutritional needs during cancer therapy, think about the following suggestions:

Suggestions

• Need to maintain good stock of foods

• Fill your fridge and pantry with healthy foods, especially those that need very little or no cooking

• Stock up foods which need less or no cooking, which can be used for emergency purpose

• Always choose small, frequent meals

• Choose healthy protein rich snacks to eat in-between i.e. peanuts, sprouts, oats etc

• Nuts, yogurt, pre-chopped veggies, and microwaveable brown rice or other whole grains are easy options

• In case of nausea/vomiting present avoid milk

• Plan a grocery list for a week

• Add healthy fruits and vegetables to your diet

During treatment

Prepare yourself to follow the diet regime throughout the treatment. In the course of cancer treatment immune system becomes weak and patient may fall sick easily. Reduced immunity results in many side effects and food borne illness too. You may have days when you feel hungry, and others when food is the last thing you want. Eat lots of protein and healthy calories. That will keep your body strong and help repair damage from the treatment. To strengthen the immunity, it is important to consume antioxidants rich fruits, vegetables, whole grains including whole wheat flour, millets, beans, eggs, fish, chicken etc. Food safety during treatment is very crucial to avoid food borne illness.

Cancerr treatment can weaken your immune system and make you more prone to infection. This includes infection from foods. The following are the tips to keep your food safe

During treatment you should also take recommendations from your doctor about what to eat and avoid.

• Selection of food quality wise;

• Choose food from a genuine source

• Avoid raw food

• Cook food at proper temperature

• Check expiry date

• Cook food until it's cooked completely or well done

• Avoid any leftover food or food from any open packet

• Keep perishable and healthy foods in fridge

• Make sure to include items you can eat even when you feel sick

• Wash vegetables or any raw foods thoroughly

• Food preparation area or chopping board should be washed thoroughly to avoid contamination

• Maintain hand hygiene (wash hand before and after eating)

• High protein and high calorie food

During cancer the body's metabolism called hypermetabolism increases that affect the requirement for high carbohydrate, protein and fat food. High calorie food includes pudding, egg nog, milkshakes, avocado, porridge pulses and legumes, curd, milk, beans, mushroom, chicken, fish and eggs etc.

Management of Side effects

Sometimes it becomes very difficult to manage the side effects,the side effects are like nausea, vomiting, diarrhea, swallowing difficulty, gastritis, taste alterations and appetite loss.

- Constipation can be avoided by adding more fluids or just plain water. High fiber foods such as vegetables, whole grains also help to prevent constipation.
- Diarrhea can be avoided by staying away from dehydration. Eat food always from a known source.
- Swallowing difficulty can be solved by including liquid foods in the daily diets. you can always choose shakes, soups or any other liquids.
- Nausea can be reduced by avoiding strong odour and spicy foods. Drink plenty of water.
- Taste alterations and appetite loss can be replenished by adding high calorie nutrient rich foods.

It can be concluded that, though you are not hungry, but you have to eat before and during your cancer treatment. Eating well with high protein and high calorie diet is important throughout the treatment to maintain the weight.Talk with your doctor, nurse, or dietitian about any eating problems that might affect you during cancer treatment. They can advise you about how to follow your special diet to cope with eating problems caused by cancer treatment.

CONCLUSION

The fact remain that, it is not possible to have "alkaline blood". The blood will naturally balance itself to remain around 7.35 to 7.45. Most studies find that eating high-alkaline foods will not increase the body's pH, nor will drinking alkaline water. Studies also have not shown a connection between an alkaline diet and a better response to chemotherapy, as some supporters claim. It is true that cancer likes acidic cell environments, but you cannot create an alkaline environment to combat cancer or become resistant to disease.

However, a low-acid diet could reduce cancer risk by helping the body naturally maintain its healthiest pH balance. You may be able to reduce your risk of cancer by eating a balanced whole-foods diet. This can enable your body to automatically correct its pH on its own, without overloading the system with acid. You do not need a special diet, but avoiding eating mostly acidic foods could prevent your body from fighting hard to achieve pH balance. This in turn can give your body its best chance at naturally preventing cancer.